How To Get The Most Out Of Your Plastic Surgery

311 Great Cosmetic Surgery Tips That You Should Follow

ADAM COLTON

Published by BizMove
www.bizmove.com

Disclaimer

All the content found in this book was created for informational purposes only. The Content is not intended to be a substitute for professional medical advice, diagnosis, or treatment. Always seek the advice of your physician or other qualified health provider with any questions you may have regarding a medical condition. Never disregard professional medical advice or delay in seeking it because of something you have read in this book.

311 Great Cosmetic Surgery Tips That You Should Follow

Surgeons can reshape the appearance of body parts through cosmetic surgery. Some of the most common body parts people want to improve through surgery include:

Breasts: Increase or reduce the size of breasts or reshape sagging breasts

Ears: Reduce the size of large ears or set protruding ears back closer to the head

Eyes: Correct drooping upper eyelids or remove puffy bags below the eyes

Face: Remove facial wrinkles, creases or acne scars

Hair: Fill in balding areas with one's own hair

Nose: Change the shape of the nose

Tummy: Flatten the abdomen

Plastic surgery is a very common procedure these days. Before you have it done, you should do your research on your surgery and find out some things on your own. The following ideas will provide you with essential information you need before having any cosmetic surgery.

1. You will probably have to remove hairs before the operation; ask your surgeon what method is best. Usually, waxing is the best solution, but you might be able to shave if you do not have a lot of hairs.

Your surgeon should be able to recommend the better method and the best products.

2. If you think, the cost of cosmetic surgery is too high in the United States, consider having the surgery done in India or Mexico. Costs are often drastically lower. You can interview doctors the same way that you would usually do, so you can expect the same level of quality work in those locations as well.

3. If you are thinking about getting some cosmetic surgery done, you need to remember that all surgery comes with risks. It does not matter how minor the surgery is, there is always the risk of complications. So remember, to be prepared for the unexpected if, you are planning some cosmetic surgery.

4. Before you see a doctor, decide what exactly you want done. Never go into a consultation without knowing precisely what you want done, because a doctor may try to convince you that you need another work done. Have a crystal clear picture in your head of what you expect, and share that with the physician during your consultation.

5. Learn about the risks of your cosmetic surgery. All surgery carries risks. Even the most routine face-lift, can result in death. Though such extreme results are

not common, it is important that you learn about all possible risks. You need to make an informed decision. Have your doctor, or surgeon explain all the risks in plain language.

6. Do not allow your child to get cosmetic surgery if they are not old enough to sign the consent forms themselves. You should let your child wait until they are fully developed both mentally and physically. Once they are of age, you can support them in whatever they choose to do.

7. Be sure to thoroughly check the qualification of your prospective surgeon. You need to research their background, education, qualifications, and disciplinary history. They have to be licensed in your area. Furthermore, be wary of doctors wanting to do complex procedure and are not surgeons. That could be a very risky gamble with your life.

8. Research the risks of the procedure(s) that you want done. Do not choose something and go into it blindly, as it could mean a great loss to your livelihood or even your life. Just like you would check side-effects with a medication, find out what could happen during surgery and after it.

9. Never get cosmetic surgery if you are going through an emotionally hard time. If you schedule it during a

stressful time, it will make your recovery more difficult and it will also intensify the stress you are experiencing. The fact that you are healing more slow may even add to the depression as well.

10.   When you are inquiring about a possible cosmetic surgery procedure, don't forget to ask about the arrangements made for anesthesia. In cosmetic surgery, anesthetization is one of the most critical (and potentially dangerous) parts of the operation. Find out who will be handling your anesthesia, and get the details on what they'll be doing.

11.   Look at the surgical center to confirm that, it has the appropriate licensing in your state. The proper accreditation assures, that the facility undergoes regular inspections. These standards reduce the risk of post-surgical infection, and other complications. If the facility does not have the proper certifications, have the procedure performed elsewhere.

12.   Learn the entire cost of your cosmetic surgery, before going under the knife. When you get your final bill, you do not want a surprise. Make sure the doctor includes not only the surgery, but any incidentals you may be billed for. Ask if, the anesthesiologist will have a separate bill.

13.   There are many minimal invasive procedures available to improve one's appearance. For example, the drug, Botox, has been shown to can help alleviate and erase the signs of aging. One of the main uses of Botox is to remove lines and wrinkles such as frown lines. The average cost for Botox treatment in the United States is around $500.00.

14.   Be comfortable when you go in for a procedure. Although cosmetic surgery is elective and relatively minor, it's still surgery. The entire process is inherently stressful. In order to minimize your stress, and make your surgery go more smoothly, take the time to familiarize yourself with the team that will be working with you. Visit the hospital, or clinic ahead of time. This way it's not an unfamiliar environment.

15.   When considering cosmetic surgery, you want to be sure that you research as much as you can about the procedure on your own. This is important, so that when you actually do talk with a professional about it the terms, and procedures that they mention are not foreign to you. That you are not hearing this information for the first time.

16.   Make sure your surgeon is certified by the American Board of Plastic Surgery. Any doctor who

has received their M.D. can legally perform cosmetic surgery. Unfortunately, cosmetic and reconstructive surgery is a very small portion of a general medicine degree. Board certified surgeons are doctors who have completed a residency in plastic surgery. They have passed several examinations to prove proficiency.

17.   Always do a lot of research about the cosmetic surgery clinics you are interested in. Make sure there have been no complaints against any of the surgeons who work there. If you find any complaints, you should find out exactly what happened and what the clinic did to make sure this wouldn't happen again.

18.   Check to see if your surgeon is qualified. When considering cosmetic surgery, you want to be sure that the surgeon you are using is competent. Check online reviews. Contact the medical board. If the surgeon is board-certified, and ask about any complaints. Checking the surgeon out now can save you a lot of grief later.

19.   Before going under the knife, always seek out a board-certified cosmetic surgeon. It is imperative that you get to know your surgeon. Ask about his qualifications, and certifications. Request before and after photos. If possible, speak with former

patients. A good surgeon will be proud to show off his best work, and will always be forthcoming about qualifications.

20.   Ask the surgeon to explain any risks that may be associated with the surgery and what can be done to minimize the risks. Research the topic by yourself to ensure your doctor's honesty; think about your surgery even more carefully when you know risks involved.

21.   If your doctor has only been talking up the benefits of your surgery, you may want to reconsider your surgeon. A quality surgeon will talk to you about not only benefits but also the risks and dangers associated with your surgery. If your doctor is nothing more than a salesman, you should keep looking.

22.   If you are thinking about getting some cosmetic surgery done, you need to remember that all surgery comes with risks. It does not matter how minor the surgery is, there is always the risk of complications. So remember, to be prepared for the unexpected if, you are planning some cosmetic surgery.

23.   Although you would never want to choose a cosmetic surgeon based solely on price, there is no harm in shopping around amongst qualified

surgeons. If you have a short list of surgeons that you are considering, discussing pricing options with each of them may help you in making the final decision.

24.   To ensure you get a good surgeon, ask where your surgeon has hospital privileges. Many surgeons practice from outpatient clinics instead of hospitals. Hospital privileges can still help potential patients determine the surgeon's credentials. Hospitals will do background checks against the surgeon's certifications, and malpractice history. Surgeons without hospital privileges need to have a good explanation for this lack.

25.   Here are four important things to consider before deciding to have cosmetic surgery. Recovery is the first item to investigate pre-surgery. Another important factor is cost and payment options. It is imperative to know what blood loss you can expect after the surgery and what antibiotics you will need to help fight off any possible infection. The risks involved in your procedure itself are also, of course, well worth investigating.

26.   Be sure to get plenty of sleep after your cosmetic procedure. Just like when you are sick, the best antidote to the post-surgery pain you may have is to sleep. Have someone else in your household

take over whatever duties you may have so you can properly rest. Turn off your phone, and shut off the lights!

27.   Be realistic in your expectations. Surgery can change your physical appearance, but there are limits to its effects. For example, if you want surgery because you suffer from low self esteem, you are probably going to continue to have low self esteem, even after your surgery. You might want to consider counseling, before you decide on surgery.

28.   Never be scared about asking questions. The doctor may use words you don't understand, so ask him to break things down for you. Ensure you understand your doctor's terminology by repeating what you understood back to him.

29.   Find someone who can stay with you for the first 24 hours, or so after surgery. While cosmetic surgery is usually relatively minor, it is still surgery. There can be complications from the anesthetic, or the surgery itself. Someone should be available to notify your doctor, in the event of any problems.

30.   Before making a decision about your plastic surgeon, ask for references. Take some time to call those references and ask them about their personal experiences. This can help you understand the

quality of work that your surgeon offers, as well as the bedside manner than he or she projects to patients. Both of these things are important and should not be taken lightly.

31.   If you want to have a cosmetic procedure done, but you don't have the money, institute a savings plan. These surgeries are scheduled many months, after you initially visit with a doctor. If you start saving a little money each week, you should be in good shape, by the time your procedure rolls around.

32.   If you want to have more than one surgery performed, talk with your doctor about the possibility of having more than one procedure done at a time. Surgeons will generally offer you substantial savings if you choose to do this. Carefully consider what your recovery time will be like. However, to make sure this is a viable option for you.

33.   Be cautious about expecting too much from your plastic surgery. While plastic surgery will change your looks, and perhaps improve your appearance, it cannot fix the problems in your life. If you are miserable before the surgery, you likely will be after as well. Expecting anything different will lead to disappointment. That is why it is

beneficial to speak with a mental health professional before, undergoing plastic surgery.

34.   Before deciding to undergo surgery, consider all other options. Sometimes there are procedures that are less-invasive and will help with your condition without surgery. You can avoid needing a cosmetic procedure by using makeup strategically, visiting your dermatologist, or using proper skin care techniques at home.

35.   You should be very cautious in selecting your cosmetic surgeon. You should talk to friends and people in your community. You should look up your surgeon online and read reviews of former patients. It is imperative that you have trust in your surgeon in order have good cosmetic surgical experience.

36.   Are you scared to get plastic surgery because of what other people will say? If you are, then it is very important to sit down with yourself. (and maybe a trusted loved one) Write down all the reasons that you are thinking about doing this. You don't need to answer to others, but you will feel more confident in your decision.

37.   Almost all reputable plastic surgeons, and their clinics have a type of computer software that allows

people to see themselves as they would look post-op. This is a great tool that should not be overlooked, as it allows you to visualize the changes you are considering. You can make a more informed decision.

38.   Discuss in detail the different kinds of procedures that the surgeon you are considering has performed in the past. Look at before and after photographs to gain a better understanding of what to expect. Although there is no step you can take to guarantee a trouble-free procedure, verifying your surgeon's expertise can really improve your odds in this respect.

39.   Talk to your surgeon about potential risks and how he or she manages those risks during surgery. Also, research your procedure so that you can confirm all of the information your doctor tells you.

40.   It is important to personally verify the medical licenses and records of doctors and hospitals or clinics you are using for your procedure. Much like you would verify a doctor's skills, you should also verify the qualifications of any potential surgery sites. This includes things such as great successes or past problems.

41.   If you are planning on having cosmetic surgery, be prepared when you meet with your surgeon. Have a list of any questions that you need answered. Ask anything, and everything that you can think of. Do not be worried about taking down some notes. It is an important decision. You might need the note later, when preparing for your surgery.

42.   Ask your surgeon if using cordran tape is a good option for you. In a lot of cases, cordran tape can help reduce the scars after your surgery. Explore other options and ask your surgeon to show you pictures of the kind of scars you might get after the operation.

43.   You should go to a different cosmetic surgeon to compare different prices and solutions. Do some research to make sure all the surgeons you go to are trustworthy. Comparing different surgeons is the best way to find the best prices and get a better idea of who is honest with you.

44.   You may be wondering what you should talk to a doctor about when it comes to plastic surgery. There are actually several bits of information you need to find out before planning any cosmetic procedure. You need to make sure they are board certified, most importantly. Ask to see pictures of patients he or she has operated on. Speak with the

surgeon about the actual surgery, medications that will be used, and the whole process of recovery.

45.   Find out from your doctor, who will be administering the anesthesia. It will either come from the surgeon, a specially-trained nurse depending on the complexity of the procedure, or an anesthesiologist. You have the right to insist that a second person administer the anesthesia as a precaution, but it will most likely cost you more.

46.   As you are visiting a surgeon for a consultation, do not become set on having a particular procedure done. An informed cosmetic surgeon will be aware of an array of options that may be appropriate in helping you achieve your desired result. Think of your surgeon as your partner, and utilize any advice they give you before you ultimately decide on your procedure.

47.   If you are considering cosmetic surgery, be sure that you are doing so at a time where you have a clear frame of mind. This is important because even though you may not realize it, times of stress can cause you to think irrationally or in a fashion that is unlike your normal thought process. Avoid making decisions like this after breakups or other emotional times.

48.   There is a good chance that you will be unhappy with the results of your cosmetic surgery. You can lessen the odds by doing your research about the surgeon and facility you are having your procedure done at. Be sure that the surgeon has all the proper certifications and a great reputation in the community.

49.   When consulting with a physician about cosmetic surgery, keep in mind that the affected area will need hair removal before the operation. Ask what method of hair removal will be used. Furthermore, think about how long it will take that hair to grow back after and what wardrobe alterations might be necessary in order to cover it up.

50.   Research the plastic surgeon. Look for recommendations and reviews from other people that have already had surgery performed by the doctor. It is best to check this out before getting the surgery done. You would not want to get a surgery performed by a doctor, who has less than perfect reviews.

51.   Ask your surgeon how many times he, or she has performed the operation you are interested in. Practice makes perfect; you should go to a surgeon who is experienced, and can show you concrete

results. A beginner might have better prices, but you should not take any risks. Go to an experienced surgeon.

52.   There are risks any time anesthesia is administered. For example, anesthesia can cause abnormal heart rhythms. Anesthesia can make your heart beat in strange ways. This happens during surgery because blood flow becomes insufficient during anesthesia. That causes a heartbeat that is irregular in pace, or arrhythmia.

53.   Before undergoing any cosmetic surgery procedure, you will want to discuss the risks and potential complications with your surgeon. Cosmetic surgeries are often elective procedures, but that certainly does not mean they are without risk. It is very important to weigh the potential benefits of the surgery against the possible complications.

54.   Speak with your insurer directly about payment for your plastic surgery procedure. While elective procedures are not typically covered, you never know until you try. Particularly, if you can prove that you need to have the procedure done for medical reasons. You may be able to receive compensation. Talk through every angle possible to see, if you can get a satisfactory answer.

55.   While the first doctor you have a consultation with may be saying all the right things, you should still talk with several more surgeons before deciding where to get the surgery done. You want to make sure that everything that is being said is true, and it is not all said just to get your business.

56.   Be sure to ask about consultation fees before you go in for your first appointment. Some surgeons charge for the office visit, but then this cost is deducted from the final price of the surgery if you choose that surgeon. Others will charge you for the visit regardless of your final choice, and some offer free consults.

57.   Before committing to undergo cosmetic surgery, see if there are non-surgical options that can improve your appearance. Cosmetic procedures normally aren't dangerous, but there can be complications. Some body issues can be remedied by a change in diet or lifestyle.

58.   Do not schedule any cosmetic procedures during an emotional time in your life. Recovering from surgery requires a great deal of energy, and emotional issues will prolong recovery and make it more difficult. Your emotional well-being can also suffer if you have a considerably slow recovery.

59.   Everything should be ready for your recovery after the surgery. Take a few weeks off work and have enough food stored in your fridge so you do not have to leave your home. Let your friends and family know you will probably need some help and might not be able to drive.

60.   There are four major things you must research before you schedule your surgery. Recovery is one of these aspects. Prices and method of payments should be your next concern. Post-op inflammation and infection is another thing to learn about. Lastly, know any other risks that have been associated with your specific procedure.

61.   Do not think that plastic surgery is the miracle cure for a lack of self-esteem. While having surgery can make you look better, it can only make you feel better if you already feel good about yourself. Go see a therapist before you go through with surgery, in order to determine if sugery is a wise choice.

62.   Find a surgeon you trust. One of the most essential elements of any successful cosmetic surgery procedure is a good surgeon. Make sure you get a chance to really talk with the doctor, before you commit to any surgery. Check online review sites, even talk with former patients if you can.

63.   If you want to have cosmetic surgery, you should investigate all the possible side effects first. There are always risks involved when you have surgery, and having cosmetic surgery is no different. The only way to make an informed decision is to know what you can expect and what might happen.

64.   A face lift, Rhytidectomy, visably improves the signs of aging in the neck, and face. For example, if a patient has lost muscle tone in the face. The patients looks as if he, or she has jowls. The average cost of a face lift surgery in the United States is a little over $5,000.00.

65.   Before you go into surgery, know what your options are if things go awry. If you do have a poor cosmetic surgery experience, you may be too emotionally compromised after the fact to effectively research your options. Do yourself the favor and do the research before hand; it can give you the peace of mind that you need to fully relax for the surgery.

66.   You are the primary decision maker in your surgery. What this means is that you should never put the opinions of others ahead of your own feelings. Even minor plastic surgeries are life-

changing events. Do not go through with a surgery if you are not certain about it.

67.   Never get plastic surgery because you feel that it will make you more attractive to someone you are interested in. While that may lead to them showing more an interest in you, the fact is that they like the image that they are seeing and not who you actually are as a person.

68.   You will probably have to remove hairs before the operation; ask your surgeon what method is best. Usually, waxing is the best solution, but you might be able to shave if you do not have a lot of hairs. Your surgeon should be able to recommend the better method and the best products.

69.   Cosmetic procedures can be quite costly, and may also require you to miss work. Because of this, it is a good idea to set aside some savings before your procedure. This helps to alleviate any worry about the financial implications of surgery.

70.   You should ask specific questions and think about certain issues when you are selecting a cosmetic surgeon. You should not select a surgeon on price alone. You will want a board-certified surgeon. You want a surgeon who takes the time to answer your questions and fears. You should trust

your instinct, if your surgeon makes your uncomfortable, you should find another one.

71.   If you have heard that someone else is getting plastic surgery, don't allow that to sway your opinion of yourself. While there are many great times to use this tool, keeping up with the Jones' is not a good enough reason. Give yourself some time to think, then reconsider the idea later on.

72.   You should keep your expectations of the results of plastic surgery realistic. Most procedures are about just an improvement over what you already look like and will not create a new face. If the procedures are centered around body contouring, remember that this is not a weight loss procedure but will merely improve the shape of your body by a few degrees.

73.   You should ask your surgeon what would happen if you were not satisfied with the results. If something went wrong during the procedure. Your surgeon should be honest with you. Let you know that you can file a claim for malpractice. If your surgeon is not honest on this topic, you should go to another clinic.

74.   Speak with your insurer directly about payment for your plastic surgery procedure. While elective

procedures are not typically covered, you never know until you try. Particularly, if you can prove that you need to have the procedure done for medical reasons. You may be able to receive compensation. Talk through every angle possible to see, if you can get a satisfactory answer.

75.   DO not think of cosmetic surgery as a game. Since, it is a serious medical procedure that can put your life at risk. Make sure to plan ahead. You can eliminate your need to have any additional surgery in the future. Know what you want, and stick with it.

76.   Liposuction is a popular cosmetic procedure. A tube is placed in through a small cut and then suction fat out. The tube goes into the fat layer, and it works to dislodge the fat cells and vacuums them out. A surgeon may use a large syringe or a vacuum pump.

77.   If you are thinking of having cosmetic surgery, make sure you know how long your recovery will be. Make plans to spend a few weeks at home; stock up on groceries and do not make any plans with your friends. You do not want to miss out on any plans because you have poor timing.

78.   Make sure you are properly prepared for eating after your cosmetic procedure. First of all, you are not going to want to eat anything too heavy, so buy light foods like soups, applesauce and Jello. Second, you probably will not have the energy to cook anything. Therefore, buy foods that can be easily made in the microwave or toaster oven.

79.   Prior to having surgery, four aspects must be thoroughly researched. Recovery is one of these aspects. Then, you might want to learn on how much it will cost you. Third, learn about inflammation and infection following the procedure. Find out what the risks are of the procedure you're interested in.

80.   When you are planning for your cosmetic surgery, do not expect the results to be perfect. Only expect an improvement from the way you looked before. If you are expecting to come through the surgery looking like your favorite model, chances are you will be let down. Keeping your expectations in check, will help you avoid depression after the procedure.

81.   Do not allow yourself to get addicted to cosmetic surgery. Once people get it done once, and are pleased with the results, they think they will look even better by continuing to get it done. Too

much plastic surgery is just going to make you look fake. It can even cause, health problems.

82.   Avoid just going with the first surgeon you meet. Take some time to speak with at least two, or three surgeons before making a final decision. Talk to some references too. This will help to ensure that you have found the most qualified surgeon for your procedure. It will also help to ensure your satisfaction in the final results.

83.   While there are no magical benefits to visualization, it can still be a helpful technique. Before you start your procedure, visualize everything going well. After you have undergone the surgery, begin to visualize a quick, complete recovery. This won't actually improve the recovery, but it will improve your state of mind.

84.   Speak with the surgeon about anything you need to do prior to having your procedure. Ask them if hair needs to be removed from your head or face.

85.   Check to see if your surgeon is qualified. When considering cosmetic surgery, you want to be sure that the surgeon you are using is competent. Check online reviews. Contact the medical board. If the surgeon is board-certified, and ask about any

complaints. Checking the surgeon out now can save you a lot of grief later.

86.   Visit the location of your surgery. If your procedure will be done on an outpatient basis in your regular doctor's office, see if you can tour the surgical rooms in advance of your operation. If you become familiar with your hospital prior to cosmetic surgery, you'll feel more comfortable.

87.   Infection normally occurs in less than one percent of surgeries. However, should you develop an infection recovery time is greatly lengthened. People who take steroids, have vascular problems, or smoke have a greater risk of infections. It has also been shown that, the length of surgery, as well as amount of blood loss increase the risk of developing an infection.

88.   Ask your surgeon if using cordran tape is a good option for you. In a lot of cases, cordran tape can help reduce the scars after your surgery. Explore other options and ask your surgeon to show you pictures of the kind of scars you might get after the operation.

89.   Before interviewing cosmetic surgeons, create a list of every question you want to ask. You need to have a good idea of a surgeon's background, and

responses to critical questions. Such as questions on complications, overall risks, and post-operative care. Have the same list handy for every interview you do. You can see how each surgeon responds, and you can make an educated choice regarding the right one for you.

90.   If you are not on vitamins, you may want to begin taking one before having the procedure done. Having any surgery done tends to deplete your body of essential nutrients and vitamins. Taking vitamins at least one month prior to surgery reduces your chances of losing an extreme amount of vitamins.

91.   If you are experiencing an emotionally driven moment in your life, do not get cosmetic surgery. Because you need energy to recover, it may be more difficult if you're emotionally unstable. Slow recovery might make your emotional health even worse.

92.   When it comes to cosmetic surgery, don't hesitate to put yourself first. This is important because your own feelings and decisions need to be a priority. Even if it's just a minor change, it takes a lot to change your appearance surgically, and it is often irreversible. Don't commit to plastic surgery unless you know that it's right for you and will help your happiness.

93. When deciding about cosmetic surgery, make sure you give yourself enough time to recover after the surgery. The body needs time to heal. You need to make sure you schedule time not only for the procedure, but time for your body to relax, and heal after the surgery is over.

94. Don't rush into any decision pertaining to cosmetic surgery. These are decisions that will physically alter your appearance and are not easily (or cheaply) undone. Any quality surgeon, will give you the time you need to make a smart decision. If you feel your surgeon is pressuring you, you may want to consider other options as there may be financial motives behind their pushiness.

95. Make sure you ask questions. Make sure you understand everything the doctor says since he will likely be using lots of complicated medical terms. Explain to the doctor that you don't understand, and ask him or her to use language that is more common.

96. Arrange alternative transport for the day of surgery and for your follow-up appointments for the next few days. Immediately, after surgery, you will be feeling the after-effects of anesthetic and be unable to drive. Furthermore, for the first few days

out of surgery, you will likely be using pain medication, which prevents you from driving.

97.   Talk to your surgeon and physician before the operation. Ask all of your questions, no matter how small or insignificant, and make sure you are satisfied with the answers. A surgeon who is willing to answer your questions will help to make your experience as smooth as possible.

98.   Ask whether your cosmetic surgery procedure will be covered by your insurance provider. Very often the answer is no, if the surgery is elective, but it is a good idea to ask anyway. They may be able to work with you to find an arrangement that you are happy with.

99.   For people who choose cosmetic surgery because of weight issues, you have to understand that it is not a cure all. It is about improvement of what the surgeon has to work with, not an extreme fix for serious weight issues. Cosmetic surgeries are most successful for those patients who have lost the majority of their weight before surgery.

100.   You may feel that cosmetic surgery is the only way to change your appearance, and appear younger. Before you go under the knife, be sure that you are 100% comfortable with your decision.

There is always a risk of becoming permanently disfigured by a botched job. Be sure that you understand not only the benefits, but the risks as well.

101.   Never get plastic surgery because you feel that it will make you more attractive to someone you are interested in. While that may lead to them showing more an interest in you, the fact is that they like the image that they are seeing and not who you actually are as a person.

102.   Make sure you understand exactly what kind of recovery period you will be after your procedure. Many people believe they can jump right back into work. While this holds true for minor surgeries, it is not possible to have a large procedure without recovery time. Talk things out with your medical professional beforehand.

103.   Cosmetic surgery is normally a lot more painful than most people expect. This is because it generally involves sensitive body parts like facial features, or breasts. It is important to consider pain management beforehand. You can implement a good strategy ,when you are actually suffering. This includes friends, and family who can take care of you.

104.   You should thoroughly research your surgeons policy on revised procedures. Surgeons have been known to mess up on a procedure, and corrective surgery can be quite expensive. Sometimes a surgeon will provide corrective surgery for free during a one year post procedure period.

105.   Find out about any potential risks associated with your type of cosmetic surgery and how your doctor would address them. Find out for yourself whether the surgeon's statements are accurate and make your decision based on all the information that you have.

106.   You should explore different alternatives to cosmetic surgery. For instance, if you are interested in changing the size of your breasts or getting a liposuction, a healthy diet and a lot of exercise could help you reach your goals and save a lot of money. Give yourself a few months to try different alternatives before getting surgery.

107.   For any cosmetic surgery, make sure that you choose a reputable cosmetic surgeon, who has the experience to do your procedure. A great surgeon will take the time to sit down with you, and help you understand the risks involved prior to having the surgery. They will also be willing to show their

credentials, and any other information that you ask for.

108.   Check for malpractice suits before you choose a surgeon. While some malpractice suits are started frivolously, a surgeon with a history of such suits is probably a poor choice. State licensing boards, and other such local certification agencies can tell you about the malpractice history of your surgeon before you commit.

109.   Although you would never want to choose a cosmetic surgeon based solely on price, there is no harm in shopping around amongst qualified surgeons. If you have a short list of surgeons that you are considering, discussing pricing options with each of them may help you in making the final decision.

110.   The most important thing to consider prior to any cosmetic procedure is whether or not you actually need the surgery. Although the majority of cosmetic surgeries have positive outcomes, these procedures are not without risk. Dissatisfaction with the results, injury or even death are all possible, so it is crucial that you are certain the potential benefits outweigh the potential risks.

111.   Do not go abroad to get surgery because of cheaper prices. Going to another country is a good option, if you have a way to make sure your surgeon is properly trained and licensed. And will perform the operation in an accredited facility. Stay away from countries where surgeons are not legally required to have a license.

112.   Don't be swayed by low rates. Quality is important, you should not just choose a surgeon because they fit into your price range. If you do, you may be unhappy with the results. You'll be forced to pay more money to get something that you don't like fixed. In addition to price, consider the qualifications of the surgeon that you are thinking about.

113.   Turning to cosmetic surgery to improve or enhance your appearance is something that should not be taken lightly. You will have to undergo some physiological testing to be sure you do not have any disorders that would make you a high-risk patient. As you are going through the testing, be sure to be completely honest to avoid any devastating outcomes once the procedure is complete.

114.   When considering cosmetic surgery, make sure that you include all of the costs involved, when checking to see whether you can fit it into your

budget. Additionally, be aware that the same procedure can cost thousands more, depending upon where you live. For example, the cost for a rhinoplasty procedure ranges from $7,000 to $13,000 in New York City. It can cost significantly less in other parts of the country.

115.   Ask yourself why you want to have cosmetic surgery. Understand that the best way for you to leave a valuable legacy in the world is by being a great parent or friend, and that does not depend on how you look. Make sure that your expectations regarding the surgery and your life afterward are realistic.

116.   Before undergoing a surgery there are several vitamins, and minerals that you need in a daily regimen. These include Vitamins A, C, and E. After you are in the recovery period, there are a few extra vitamins. B6 and B12 that you will want to add to the previous ones.

117.   Always do a lot of research about the cosmetic surgery clinics you are interested in. Make sure there have been no complaints against any of the surgeons who work there. If you find any complaints, you should find out exactly what happened and what the clinic did to make sure this wouldn't happen again.

118.   If you have already decided on one surgery or another, and it is coming soon, there is some preparing you need to do. One of the most important things to consider is your pre-op diet. You want to avoid gaining or losing too much weight in this period as it can change things for your doctor.

119.   When looking at any type of surgery, you should always be prepared for problems. This is even more true with plastic surgery, as you also have the chance of a botched job. This isn't meant to scare you off, just as a reminder to have the number of a back-up surgeon on hand.

120.   You should ask your surgeon what would happen if you were not satisfied with the results. If something went wrong during the procedure. Your surgeon should be honest with you. Let you know that you can file a claim for malpractice. If your surgeon is not honest on this topic, you should go to another clinic.

121.   If your doctor has only been talking up the benefits of your surgery, you may want to reconsider your surgeon. A quality surgeon will talk to you about not only benefits but also the risks and dangers associated with your surgery. If your doctor

is nothing more than a salesman, you should keep looking.

122. Before undergoing any cosmetic surgery procedure, you will want to discuss the risks and potential complications with your surgeon. Cosmetic surgeries are often elective procedures, but that certainly does not mean they are without risk. It is very important to weigh the potential benefits of the surgery against the possible complications.

123. Consider having cosmetic surgery overseas. Cosmetic surgery in the United States can cost double, or triple the amount you would be charged in India. Doctors in many countries are just as well trained as U.S. doctors, sometimes more so. Research the clinic, and doctor you plan to use, either in the U.S. or overseas.

124. Ask your surgeon if using cordran tape is a good option for you. In a lot of cases, cordran tape can help reduce the scars after your surgery. Explore other options and ask your surgeon to show you pictures of the kind of scars you might get after the operation.

125. Even if your surgeon suggests multiple procedures, consider having just one surgery done

at a time. The more surgeries that are performed at the same time, the higher the risk for complications and errors. Having multiple surgeries at the same time means you as the patient are under anaesthetic for a longer time, which carries its own set of risks.

126.   Liposuction is a popular cosmetic procedure. A tube is placed in through a small cut and then suction fat out. The tube goes into the fat layer, and it works to dislodge the fat cells and vacuums them out. A surgeon may use a large syringe or a vacuum pump.

127.   Your cosmetic surgeon will make decisions that you must respect. If a surgeon tells you not to have a particular surgery done, there's more than likely a reason as to why. If you truly don't agree, ask another surgeon what they think. Most surgeons have their patients' safety in mind; therefore, you should follow your surgeons advice.

128.   If your teenager is asking for cosmetic surgery, you should wait until he or she is done growing and is mature enough to make an educated decision. Offering the child the opportunity to alter their appearance can be good for their self-esteem, but keep in mind that their body will probably keep changing after the surgery.

129.   Getting cosmetic surgery is not cheap, and it's definitely one of the things that your health insurance won't reimburse you for. There is a different fee for each kind of surgery. Before you go into surgery, make sure you can handle the cost of it. As you add up the cost of the whole process, make sure to add in post-op costs and any future procedures.

130.   A good cosmetic surgeon understands, that despite all mental preparation prior to a surgery, a patient is still going to have fears and concerns, after the surgical procedure is complete. You should feel at ease in contacting your surgeon post surgery, to discuss these concerns and worries.

131.   If your procedure involves lasers, you need to find out how experienced your surgeon is. You should never opt for laser surgery which will not be done by a physician. While some facilities may permit other medical personnel to operate the lasers, it is best to have a licensed physician perform your procedure.

132.   Find someone who can stay with you for the first 24 hours, or so after surgery. While cosmetic surgery is usually relatively minor, it is still surgery. There can be complications from the anesthetic, or

the surgery itself. Someone should be available to notify your doctor, in the event of any problems.

133.   Expect some scarring. Many people go into cosmetic surgery with unrealistic expectations of emerging with a perfect body. While many procedures have made advancements towards minimizing this, the fact remains that most leave some sort of scar. Tummy tucks are among the largest, and you can expect a permanent scar from hip to hip after surgery.

134.   When looking at any type of cosmetic surgery, you should be sure to shop around. People who undergo surgery without first doing so are often more likely to suffer from a poor-quality surgeon. Talk to at least 4 or 5 professionals before closing your surgery in order to ensure quality.

135.   You should consider the following when you are considering a tummy tuck. To be a good candidate for this type of procedure, you should be close to optimum body weight. You might have some loose skin around the belly area caused by pregnancy, or rapid weight loss. A cosmetic surgeon will want you to be at your ideal weight, in order to have a successful procedure.

136.   Before going under the knife, always seek out a board-certified cosmetic surgeon. It is imperative that you get to know your surgeon. Ask about his qualifications, and certifications. Request before and after photos. If possible, speak with former patients. A good surgeon will be proud to show off his best work, and will always be forthcoming about qualifications.

137.   Cosmetic surgery should always undergone with a sound mind. This means you need to check out as much, as you can about the surgeon beforehand. Don't worry about being offensive when you ask him personal questions about his qualifications. Include the school, and extra courses that he has studied. This helps give you peace of mind.

138.   Take the time to go over prices with your surgeon and ask him or her to break down the final prices for you. Set a date for the final payment, and see if it is possible to build a payment plan. In order to keep issues from arising later on, come to a consensus with your surgeon about payment before you undergo the procedure.

139.   Prevent complications from cosmetic surgery by eating a nutritious diet and using vitamin supplements when you can. Surgery is always something that takes time to get over, but you need

to prepare yourself to recover by making sure your body can do the work it needs to do. Proper nutrition will help.

140.   If your doctor has only been talking up the benefits of your surgery, you may want to reconsider your surgeon. A quality surgeon will talk to you about not only benefits but also the risks and dangers associated with your surgery. If your doctor is nothing more than a salesman, you should keep looking.

141.   Ask your surgeon if he will be handling anesthesia for your cosmetic surgery alone. If so, insist on having an anesthesiologist, or anesthesiology nurse participate in your surgery. If there is a problem with anesthesia during the surgery, the doctor may have difficulty dealing with both the anesthesia, and the surgery.

142.   You need to feel totally comfortable with any cosmetic surgeon that you decide on.

143.   You need to absolutely trust them and feel at ease when you are having any discussions with them. You are trusting them with your body and potentially your life, so you have to feel at ease when you are with them.

144.   Schedule a decent amount of recovery time following any cosmetic surgery. Healing time is needed for your body after any surgery. So clear your schedule, and give your body the proper time to heal. Don't be tempted to return to work too early. You may be feeling better now, but after strenuous activity, you may realize your body is not yet ready to take on the work day.

145.   You should go to a different cosmetic surgeon to compare different prices and solutions. Do some research to make sure all the surgeons you go to are trustworthy. Comparing different surgeons is the best way to find the best prices and get a better idea of who is honest with you.

146.   Find a surgeon you trust. One of the most essential elements of any successful cosmetic surgery procedure is a good surgeon. Make sure you get a chance to really talk with the doctor, before you commit to any surgery. Check online review sites, even talk with former patients if you can.

147.   Be sure to verify the qualifications of your surgeon when it comes to your specific procedure. You need to also make sure that the surgeon's license is not expired. You could do this by asking and inquiring from the state's licensing bureau. Not

only will it build your confidence in your surgeon, it is also free of charge to investigate.

148.   Depending on the type of cosmetic surgery you are undergoing, you are going to have to allow for the appropriate time to heal. Some surgeries only require a few days, while others can require you to rest for many weeks. Know that you may be out of work for a while and not able to care for things around the home until you are fully healed.

149.   A cosmetic surgery to correct a nose is called rhinoplasty. Many of today's teens request a nose job to create the perfect nose. You may wish to consider having rhinoplasty for your teen if his, or her nose has been broken. The average cost for rhinoplasty in the United States is approximately $4,000.00. While this procedure seems high, the advantages of your teen's self esteem is worth it.

150.   If cosmetic surgery seems out of your price range, you can consider getting it done outside of the United States. Medical tourism has exploded in popularity, as the costs associated with certain procedures are sometimes half the price in a foreign country. But be careful with who you choose to do the procedure. Do your research into the surgeon's credentials prior to signing on the bottom line.

151.   Do not get cosmetic surgery from a surgeon whom you have not checked out. You want to make sure that your surgery goes well, and that the surgeon who is conducting the surgery on you is trustworthy. You can ask previous patients to figure out if the doctor is reliable or not.

152.   Make sure you do a little research on cosmetic surgery before you go under the knife. You are going to want to understand all that is involved with cosmetic surgery like costs, risks, and how you should prepare for the actual surgery. After a little research you can determine if cosmetic surgery is for you or not.

153.   Always ask your surgeon about his or her credentials and do some research yourself. Ask what school he went to, when he graduated, as well as how many procedures has he done. Definitely ask to see success photographs of past patients.

154.   Make sure you do your research about any surgeon whom you are considering. Take a look at where they went to school and investigate whether they have received any awards or been disciplined in any way. It is impossible to make an educated decision about which surgeon to use unless you take these factors into consideration.

155.   You can take steps to save money on your cosmetic surgery procedure without skimping. Some other countries offer reputable doctors while saving you a lot of money. This is something to take into consideration, even though it may not always be an option.

156.   Make sure to review the credentials for the location where your surgery will take place. You don't want to go to a medical facility that you haven't checked out first, so do your homework in advance. Don't forget to look at problems and success from past cases.

157.   Choose a cosmetic surgeon whom you feel comfortable with and trust. Even if a surgeon gets favorable reviews from your friends, if you do not feel relaxed with the person, you should go in another direction. Cosmetic surgery is stressful as it is; you need a doctor that you feel can offer you the support that you need.

158.   Prior to getting cosmetic surgery, be aware that there may be complications from the procedure. Your plastic surgeon will more than likely go over these potential complications with you. It is important for you to be aware of them. Some of the complications may include infection, swelling,

increased blood pressure, and although rare, even death.

159.   If you are planning on having cosmetic surgery, be prepared when you meet with your surgeon. Have a list of any questions that you need answered. Ask anything, and everything that you can think of. Do not be worried about taking down some notes. It is an important decision. You might need the note later, when preparing for your surgery.

160.   Use cosmetic surgery as a last resort when dealing with your appearance issues. Most procedures go well, but there are a lot of risks you need to consider. You can avoid these risks by choosing alternatives; any procedure related to weight can be replaced by a healthier lifestyle for instance.

161.   Ask about charges for follow-up appointments to check on your healing status. Your surgeon should offer some number of follow-up appointments as part of the cost of the surgery. Generally, follow-up appointments and consults to determine the need for revisions are free inside of the first year after the procedure.

162.   Find out if the procedure you want, requires anesthesia. The types are either local, general, or

semi-conscious sedation. Talk about the risk and safety of each one with your physician prior to getting your procedure. Many procedures allow you to choose, but general sedation tends to be more expensive. Furthermore, be sure to ask how much you will need and what they will do if it's not enough for you.

163.   Give yourself sufficient recovery time after your surgery is completed. It is possible that your recovery could take as much as four weeks, depending on the type of cosmetic surgery you have. If you have a job, take enough time off. Also, don't try to push yourself too fast.

164.   Before you even have your cosmetic procedure done, it may be wise to get yourself some stool softeners. Many people experience major constipation when they have any procedure done. Plastic surgeries are no exception. Being constipated is not good for your health, a stool softener can be of great assistance.

165.   Talk to friends and family, about your surgery. Let them know what procedure is being done, and what your recovery time will be like. If you need them to help you in any way. That way, everyone knows what to expect. You can minimize any drama before it happens.

166.   Find out what type of anesthesia will be used for the procedure and who will be administering it. Make certain that you understand the potential side effects. You should also confirm the credentials of those involved. By doing your research, you will know how to prepare for your post-surgical time.

167.   Give some thought to after the surgery. You will be extremely glad to have some advanced plans set up after you get major cosmetic work done, like a tummy tuck, a breast augmentation, or rhinoplasty. The recovery time can be rough for these major surgical procedures, so always plan in advance. Before you have your procedure, take off time from work to recover afterward, and consider having a friend help you with chores around the house.

168.   Check the plastic surgeon's education out. If you are considering any type of cosmetic surgery, you will want to make sure it is done correctly. It is best to research the education the doctor has received and make sure they are licensed before making the decision to have them perform your surgery.

169.   After you get cosmetic surgery make sure that you do not touch your face for a while. Even if your face may feel itchy, or you may want to touch it, try to let it heal as much as possible. You do not want

to mess anything up so leave your face alone for a little while.

170.   Always make sure that you meet the surgeon who will be administering your procedure ahead of time. In many cases, the only people, you come in contact with are counselors and nurses. Do not settle with that: Insist that you would like to meet the surgeon who will be in charge. You should choose another surgeon if your request is not granted.

171.   Investigate whether or not the surgeon has a license. Also, look to see whether, or not the person you are considering is board certified, or not. While neither of these things guarantees that your surgery will be performed without error. Generally surgeons with these qualifications, are more experienced in their field.

172.   The use of anesthesia is an important part of your surgery and has risks associated with it. Anesthesia can cause you to develop an abnormal heart rhythm during the procedure. General anesthesia can sometimes cause irregular heart beats. The blood flow slows down due to the anesthetic, and this affects the beating of your heart. Because of this, irregular heart beat, or arrhythmia occurs.

173.   After you receive Botox injections, do not feel alarmed, or upset of you do not see any noticeable changes in your face right after the procedure is done. In many cases, it can take up to an entire week, before you start to see the full effects of it.

174.   Investigate your cosmetic surgeon's case load before scheduling procedures with him. Although the most expert surgeons keep their schedules very busy, you want to watch out for the signs of overwork. You deserve personalized attention. Make sure that the doctor you pick out has the time to give it to you.

175.   Learn the entire cost of your cosmetic surgery, before going under the knife. When you get your final bill, you do not want a surprise. Make sure the doctor includes not only the surgery, but any incidentals you may be billed for. Ask if, the anesthesiologist will have a separate bill.

176.   A good cosmetic surgeon understands, that despite all mental preparation prior to a surgery, a patient is still going to have fears and concerns, after the surgical procedure is complete. You should feel at ease in contacting your surgeon post surgery, to discuss these concerns and worries.

177.   When you are changing your diet to prepare for an upcoming surgery, there are a few things you want to consider. While what you eat is the most important, you can fine-tune your body through supplements and vitamins. For women, it is important to ingest vitamins like C, A, and E.

178.   While you may be a good parent and have some well-behaved kids. You may want to see if a relative can watch, then for a few days after surgery. It will be hard for you to cook for them and take care of them while you are trying to recover.

179.   You must prepare yourself about a month before cosmetic surgery. You especially need to avoid the use of pain kills. You really need to avoid using them for the first month if at all possible. The reason for this is that pain killers, because they thin your blood, can reduce your skin's ability to heal itself.

180.   Prior to undergoing any cosmetic surgery, be sure to ask your surgeon about his certifications. The list of certifications he holds should include The American Board of Plastic Surgery. If he does not hold that certification, move on to another surgeon. Do not be fooled, by certificates that do not hold the high standards that this one does.

181.   Before having cosmetic surgery, ask yourself how you expect to feel once the surgery is done. Are you having surgery because of an issue that makes you life more difficult, or are you expecting to increase your self esteem? There is not necessarily a wrong answer, but you should adjust your expectations accordingly.

182.   Be cautious about expecting too much from your plastic surgery. While plastic surgery will change your looks, and perhaps improve your appearance, it cannot fix the problems in your life. If you are miserable before the surgery, you likely will be after as well. Expecting anything different will lead to disappointment. That is why it is beneficial to speak with a mental health professional before, undergoing plastic surgery.

183.   Prior to your cosmetic surgery procedure, there are many things you can do make your recovery process easier. Fill up the car with gas, water your plants, clean the house, do your grocery shopping, wash your laundry. Also, have plenty of easy-to-prepare meals, and snacks on hand. Taking care of all of these things in the days preceding your surgery, can make your recovery a whole lot more comfortable.

184.   You may feel that cosmetic surgery is the only way to change your appearance, and appear younger. Before you go under the knife, be sure that you are 100% comfortable with your decision. There is always a risk of becoming permanently disfigured by a botched job. Be sure that you understand not only the benefits, but the risks as well.

185.   Make sure you understand exactly what kind of recovery period you will be after your procedure. Many people believe they can jump right back into work. While this holds true for minor surgeries, it is not possible to have a large procedure without recovery time. Talk things out with your medical professional beforehand.

186.   When contemplating cosmetic procedures requiring surgery, it is wise to request a fair number of before and after photographs prior to scheduling your operation. By assessing the true potential as well as the limitations of your chosen procedure, you will head into the process with realistic expectations of what is achievable, thereby avoiding possible disappointment.

187.   Make sure you do your research about any surgeon whom you are considering. Take a look at where they went to school and investigate whether

they have received any awards or been disciplined in any way. It is impossible to make an educated decision about which surgeon to use unless you take these factors into consideration.

188.   Investigate whether or not the surgeon has a license. Also, look to see whether, or not the person you are considering is board certified, or not. While neither of these things guarantees that your surgery will be performed without error. Generally surgeons with these qualifications, are more experienced in their field.

189.   Ask your surgeon how many times he, or she has performed the operation you are interested in. Practice makes perfect; you should go to a surgeon who is experienced, and can show you concrete results. A beginner might have better prices, but you should not take any risks. Go to an experienced surgeon.

190.   There are many clinics that perform the surgery, but then they act as if they do not want to be bothered with you once it is over. Make sure that the clinic you have scheduled your surgery with provides after care visits for patients if something goes wrong.

191.   Learn about any financing that is available to you. You can arrange a prepayment plan with most doctors for whatever procedure you are going to have performed. If the doctor cannot help, look into other financing options so that you don't have to pay the entire cost upfront.

192.   Ask about different options for the anesthesia. For major interventions, a general anesthesia is best, but you should know about the risks involved. You have the right to ask for a general or a local anesthesia but do more research so you can make an educated decision. Ask your surgeon to have a qualified nurse assists him or her for the anesthesia if necessary.

193.   Not only should you research your specific surgeon, but you should also research the hospital or clinic at which you'll have your procedure. Any business who handles plastic surgery must follow the law. They need a proper business license, and they must be fully accredited. Even physician surgeons need to be inspected and registered as well. Make sure that your surgery center is licensed. It also needs to have a positive record.

194.   For any cosmetic surgery, make sure that you choose a reputable cosmetic surgeon, who has the experience to do your procedure. A great surgeon

will take the time to sit down with you, and help you understand the risks involved prior to having the surgery. They will also be willing to show their credentials, and any other information that you ask for.

195.   In addition to knowing about the different types of anesthesia available, it is also important to know how it will be applied. Surgeons are allowed to give general or local doses, but for more complicated procedures, a specialist will be brought in. This will affect the overall cost as well as quality of the procedure.

196.   Do not think that plastic surgery is the miracle cure for a lack of self-esteem. While having surgery can make you look better, it can only make you feel better if you already feel good about yourself. Go see a therapist before you go through with surgery, in order to determine if sugery is a wise choice.

197.   Keep the area of your incision clean after your cosmetic procedure. Just like with any other surgery you may have, cleaning the incision site is important, as it prevents infection. Once the site has healed, you may even want to consider using cocoa butter on it to help fade the appearance of a scar.

198.   Check out the malpractice history of any surgeon you are considering. While most doctors have had malpractice claims filed against them, do not deal with any surgeon who has an excessive amount. That would be a sure way to put your life at risk. It is not worth it since, there are plenty of other surgeons to choose from.

199.   If you are considering a cosmetic surgery procedure, perhaps you should be open to the idea of traveling. Although you may be able to find a good surgeon locally, especially for more common procedures, he or she may not be as experienced as surgeons in areas. Where elective cosmetic procedures are more common.

200.   When considering cosmetic surgery, be sure that you get outside opinions on whether or not you should have it. This is important because a lot of times, it does take an outside opinion to help you make your final decision. Sometimes it takes fresh eyes to see the most important points.

201.   After you get cosmetic surgery make sure that you do not touch your face for a while. Even if your face may feel itchy, or you may want to touch it, try to let it heal as much as possible. You do not want to mess anything up so leave your face alone for a little while.

202.   Cosmetic surgery should always undergone with a sound mind. This means you need to check out as much, as you can about the surgeon beforehand. Don't worry about being offensive when you ask him personal questions about his qualifications. Include the school, and extra courses that he has studied. This helps give you peace of mind.

203.   Also go over surgery costs with your surgeon, and ask to have the final prices broken down for you. Discuss the payment, and establish a plan if one is needed. Make sure that you reach a payment agreement with your doctor before surgery to avoid problems later.

204.   Remember to do a lot of research when it comes to choosing a plastic surgeon. Selecting the wrong physician can have potentially dangerous results. Inquire of family and friends as to whether they know of a plastic surgeon that they can recommend.

205.   Be aware of the risks involved with any kind of surgical procedure. Ask the physician what negative outcomes could arise as a result of the procedure. It is common to overlook the potential risks when considering plastic surgery.

206.   It is not uncommon to lose blood after having an operation. Most surgeries involve some bleeding, but too much blood loss can cause severe problems. It can occur while the surgery is happening, or after. If excessive bleeding occurs after surgery, blood will pool under the skin resulting in additional surgery to correct the issue. Talk with your doctor about what to expect after surgery.

207.   Choose a cosmetic surgeon whom you feel comfortable with and trust. Even if a surgeon gets favorable reviews from your friends, if you do not feel relaxed with the person, you should go in another direction. Cosmetic surgery is stressful as it is; you need a doctor that you feel can offer you the support that you need.

208.   DO not think of cosmetic surgery as a game. Since, it is a serious medical procedure that can put your life at risk. Make sure to plan ahead. You can eliminate your need to have any additional surgery in the future. Know what you want, and stick with it.

209.   Schedule a decent amount of recovery time following any cosmetic surgery. Healing time is needed for your body after any surgery. So clear your schedule, and give your body the proper time to heal. Don't be tempted to return to work too

early. You may be feeling better now, but after strenuous activity, you may realize your body is not yet ready to take on the work day.

210.   Before deciding to turn to plastic surgery, see if you can fix whatever you are unhappy with. While cosmetic surgery is usually very safe, there is still that small chance that something can go seriously wrong. Some common complaints, including obesity, can be treated in other ways.

211.   Talk to your doctor about complications and risks. Make sure you understand everyone. It can be easy to be so excited that you do not consider risks or complications to your cosmetic surgery, but you have to know that they exist. Listen to your doctor and determine how you can avoid both.

212.   If you are not ready for plastic surgery, wait. Many types of cosmetic surgery are simple and can be performed quickly. This can often times talk people into making hasty decisions. Stay in control of the decision- it's yours to make. Take your time, too!

213.   Make sure your surgeon is certified by the American Board of Plastic Surgery. Any doctor who has received their M.D. can legally perform cosmetic surgery. Unfortunately, cosmetic and

reconstructive surgery is a very small portion of a general medicine degree. Board certified surgeons are doctors who have completed a residency in plastic surgery. They have passed several examinations to prove proficiency.

214.   Look into getting a credit card that is specifically for health care. This type of card is just for medical procedures. You pay off a portion of what you owe each month, just like with a regular credit card. They make paying for the procedure easier, although you need to make sure you will be able to afford the payments, or you could wind up owing a lot of money.

215.   If you are finding that more and more wrinkles are creeping up onto your face and creams, and anti-aging lotions are not doing the trick, you may want to consider Botox injections. Botox injections are a painless and quick procedure to reduce immediately the appearance of your wrinkles. The injections do not cause scarring, and your face will look rejuvenated in no time!

216.   While diet is always important, it should be maintained throughout your life. It is especially important around one month before a cosmetic surgery. A proper diet means, that your body is better prepared to heal itself in the recovery period.

Avoid fried, or fatty foods. Stick with healthy whole carbs, and proteins.

217.   Do ask your doctor if the cosmetic surgery you are considering will run the risk of scarring, or infection. Some surgeries are always going to leave a scar. Although in some cases, the scar might be preferable to the current reality. Always assess the risk of infection. Also, consider how dangerous the possible infections can be.

218.   You should consider the following when you are considering a tummy tuck. To be a good candidate for this type of procedure, you should be close to optimum body weight. You might have some loose skin around the belly area caused by pregnancy, or rapid weight loss. A cosmetic surgeon will want you to be at your ideal weight, in order to have a successful procedure.

219.   When contemplating cosmetic procedures requiring surgery, it is wise to request a fair number of before and after photographs prior to scheduling your operation. By assessing the true potential as well as the limitations of your chosen procedure, you will head into the process with realistic expectations of what is achievable, thereby avoiding possible disappointment.

220.   When looking at any type of surgery, you should always be prepared for problems. This is even more true with plastic surgery, as you also have the chance of a botched job. This isn't meant to scare you off, just as a reminder to have the number of a back-up surgeon on hand.

221.   Before interviewing cosmetic surgeons, create a list of every question you want to ask. You need to have a good idea of a surgeon's background, and responses to critical questions. Such as questions on complications, overall risks, and post-operative care. Have the same list handy for every interview you do. You can see how each surgeon responds, and you can make an educated choice regarding the right one for you.

222.   Think about paying for your procedure in cash. Surgeons are often stuck with large provider fees resulting from third-party financing; as a result, you pay more. Talk with your doctor about any savings that may result from you choosing this method of payment. There are also websites available, that can show you your options based on which doctor you choose.

223.   One of the main reasons people have cosmetic surgery is to increase their self-esteem. People who have gone though a major injury, like a burn, can

really benefit from it. Sometimes people are involved in accidents that require extensive plastic surgery to repair burned tissue. This plastic surgery is necessary so the person can feel whole and improve their self esteem.

224.   When considering cosmetic surgery, it is crucial that you ask questions about your recovery time, and any post-op care that you will need. You might need time to recover after surgery. Be aware of the length of your recovery ahead of time to avoid hurting yourself.

225.   If you are having emotional problems right now, don't go for cosmetic surgery until you are feeling better. When you have emotional stress factors to worry about, it can be extremely difficult to get through surgery and the recovery process in a healthy, timely manner. The slower your recovery, the worse you may end up feeling emotionally.

226.   Before you need it, raise as much of the money as you can for your cosmetic surgery. While there are pricing options available to you, they often have interest rates that you can avoid. To avoid high financing fees, simply take the time to raise your own money before the surgery.

227.   Find out if the procedure you want, requires anesthesia. The types are either local, general, or semi-conscious sedation. Talk about the risk and safety of each one with your physician prior to getting your procedure. Many procedures allow you to choose, but general sedation tends to be more expensive. Furthermore, be sure to ask how much you will need and what they will do if it's not enough for you.

228.   Investigate every doctor you consult with, for any malpractice suits. This is fairly simple to do. Every state has an Office of Insurance Regulation, so make sure to check this out before you have your surgery. You don't want to end up seeing a doctor who has a history of malpractice suits.

229.   If cosmetic surgery is in your plans you need to be sure to eat well before, during, and after. Eating properly will help you to get through the surgery safely. It will also help you when you are recovering after. Drinking enough water is also important, and should not be forgotten.

230.   It is easy to overlook the importance of eating healthy foods when considering cosmetic surgery. Properly eaten fats are an essential macronutrient for a prepartory diet. When you are preparing for

surgery, fats from foods like avocado and flax oil should be eaten.

231.   Do ask your doctor if the cosmetic surgery you are considering will run the risk of scarring, or infection. Some surgeries are always going to leave a scar. Although in some cases, the scar might be preferable to the current reality. Always assess the risk of infection. Also, consider how dangerous the possible infections can be.

232.   While there are no magical benefits to visualization, it can still be a helpful technique. Before you start your procedure, visualize everything going well. After you have undergone the surgery, begin to visualize a quick, complete recovery. This won't actually improve the recovery, but it will improve your state of mind.

233.   Before you decide on getting surgery or not, do as much research as possible. One important area to consider carefully is how much the surgery will cost, and what you will do to pay for it. How much is it going to cost? Do not forget to take post-op care and visits to the surgeon into consideration.

234.   Confirm with your doctor how long you are going to have to be on antibiotics for after surgery. Antibiotics can make you feel a bit different, and

not function properly. So you are going to want to know how long it is going to take, before you fully recover. Then you can live a normal life again.

235.   Before deciding on a surgeon, find out if they warranty their services. There have been times where surgeons have done bad procedures and the patient had to pay a lot of money in order to get things corrected. Ask your surgeon if he provides corrective surgeries that are free of cost.

236.   If you have heard that someone else is getting plastic surgery, don't allow that to sway your opinion of yourself. While there are many great times to use this tool, keeping up with the Jones' is not a good enough reason. Give yourself some time to think, then reconsider the idea later on.

237.   Cosmetic surgery should always undergone with a sound mind. This means you need to check out as much, as you can about the surgeon beforehand. Don't worry about being offensive when you ask him personal questions about his qualifications. Include the school, and extra courses that he has studied. This helps give you peace of mind.

238.   There are many clinics that perform the surgery, but then they act as if they do not want to be bothered with you once it is over. Make sure that

the clinic you have scheduled your surgery with provides after care visits for patients if something goes wrong.

239.   Almost all cosmetic surgeons will have a book available for their previous jobs, even for intimate changes such as breast surgery. Be sure to ask to take a look at this book so you can see the level of success your doctor has experienced in the past. This also gives you a chance to make detailed decisions about your own changes.

240.   Before you got your surgery, you almost certainly looked at a before, and after book to make an informed decision. Be sure to pass this favor on. Even if you feel uncomfortable about showing your body. This will help other people to make an informed decision about their own surgery.

241.   DO not think of cosmetic surgery as a game. Since, it is a serious medical procedure that can put your life at risk. Make sure to plan ahead. You can eliminate your need to have any additional surgery in the future. Know what you want, and stick with it.

242.   Do not be afraid to ask your plastic surgeon anything you want to ask. Many people feel that their questions are silly, and refrain from asking

them. As a patient, it is your right to know everything that is going on with your health. No matter what it is, ask your plastic surgeon!

243.   Many cosmetic surgeons, and clinics specialize on relatively narrow areas. Sometimes they concentrate on just one procedure. You should look for a doctor with a broader view. A good specialist in cosmetic work should, be able to help guide you to procedures that really solve your problems. Someone who does all kinds of surgery will be able to present you with more options.

244.   Make sure you are properly prepared for eating after your cosmetic procedure. First of all, you are not going to want to eat anything too heavy, so buy light foods like soups, applesauce and Jello. Second, you probably will not have the energy to cook anything. Therefore, buy foods that can be easily made in the microwave or toaster oven.

245.   Before you go into surgery, know what your options are if things go awry. If you do have a poor cosmetic surgery experience, you may be too emotionally compromised after the fact to effectively research your options. Do yourself the favor and do the research before hand; it can give you the peace of mind that you need to fully relax for the surgery.

246.   Whatever procedure you decide on, it is vital that you choose a surgeon who is properly qualified for that particular surgery. You don't want to use a surgeon with an expired license, so make sure it is current. This can easily be accomplished by ringing up the licensing bureau. State licensing bureaus don't charge you anything to confirm licenses, and it will help increase your confidence in the surgeon to double check.

247.   Check out the malpractice history of any surgeon you are considering. While most doctors have had malpractice claims filed against them, do not deal with any surgeon who has an excessive amount. That would be a sure way to put your life at risk. It is not worth it since, there are plenty of other surgeons to choose from.

248.   Plan so that your life is not overly demanding for the two weeks immediately after your surgery. When you consider cosmetic surgery, it is not as simple as taking a day off, and then going right back to work. Factor in recovery time. Also as having someone available to help you if, you need assistance for a few days.

249.   Find out how long it will take you to recover after the surgery. Ask about how much pain you

should expect. Perhaps you should take painkillers, or plan on spending a few days in bed after your surgery. Make all the arrangements necessary before, going to surgery if you should expect a long recovery.

250.   Almost all reputable plastic surgeons, and their clinics have a type of computer software that allows people to see themselves as they would look post-op. This is a great tool that should not be overlooked, as it allows you to visualize the changes you are considering. You can make a more informed decision.

251.   One important aspect of surgeon research prior to cosmetic surgery is an investigation of the surgeon's malpractice history. You want to know if he or she has had any claims filed against him or her. Although any surgeon may end up with a dissatisfied patient, multiple claims would be a big red flag.

252.   During your pre-surgery consultation with your cosmetic surgeon, you will want to discuss anesthesia. It is important to know that a qualified anesthetist will be administering your anesthesia, and monitoring your health during the procedure. You will also want to discuss the various anesthesia options that are available to you.

253.   Learn of what preparations you will need to take for surgery after-care. Certain cosmetic surgeries, such as breast augmentation, require you to take medications, or creams after you have the procedure. It is wise to learn about after-care before surgery. The last thing you want to have to do after the procedure, is run out to get the products.

254.   One important thing to do when considering cosmetic surgery is, to make sure that you check around, and compare potential surgeons. You will find that it well worth your while, to make sure that you find one that will let you know of potential risks, and also one that you feel the most comfortable with.

255.   If your teenager is asking for cosmetic surgery, you should wait until he or she is done growing and is mature enough to make an educated decision. Offering the child the opportunity to alter their appearance can be good for their self-esteem, but keep in mind that their body will probably keep changing after the surgery.

256.   If you are having difficulty finding a doctor that is affordable, think about going to another city to have your chosen procedure done. The cost of a surgery can range depending on where it is

performed, so you can usually get what you want within your price range if you are willing to travel. Make sure to compare the potential savings to the cost of the travel to make sure that it is worth it.

257.   Be sure to ask whether your plastic surgeon is a cosmetic surgeon, or a reconstructive surgeon. While the two sub-specialties both fall under the umbrella of plastic surgery. They can be very different in practice. If you are seeking cosmetic surgery, you want a surgeon familiar with cosmetic surgery in general, and the procedure you seek specifically.

258.   There are many minimal invasive procedures available to improve one's appearance. For example, the drug, Botox, has been shown to can help alleviate and erase the signs of aging. One of the main uses of Botox is to remove lines and wrinkles such as frown lines. The average cost for Botox treatment in the United States is around $500.00.

259.   Make sure you have realistic hopes for your procedure's outcome. Cosmetic surgery can transform you, but there are limits, risks and a new appearance will not transform your life. That is particularly the case if you have existing psychological factors that affect your body image. Simply changing physical appearance might not be

sufficient for relieving your personal issues. You should find a specialist who understands your situation.

260.   You may have some sort of conflict with your surgeon because they refuse to do a procedure for you. There is probably a good reason for this, and they are looking out for your best interests, so listen to them. If you want, look to another doctor for a second opinion.

261.   Don't rush into any decision pertaining to cosmetic surgery. These are decisions that will physically alter your appearance and are not easily (or cheaply) undone. Any quality surgeon, will give you the time you need to make a smart decision. If you feel your surgeon is pressuring you, you may want to consider other options as there may be financial motives behind their pushiness.

262.   It is very important that you drink enough water at all times. This is especially important when your body undergoes extreme stress, such as a surgical procedure. For at least six weeks before your surgery, and for several months afterwards, drink lots of water. Carry a water bottle and keep it filled.

263.   Learn about the kind of anesthesia that will be used. General and IV sedation are commonly used

for more complicated and bigger surgeries. Smaller more localized procedures will only require the use of a local anesthetic. Understanding, which will be used in your case will help you understand the cost and the risks you are facing.

264.   Research the plastic surgeon. Look for recommendations and reviews from other people that have already had surgery performed by the doctor. It is best to check this out before getting the surgery done. You would not want to get a surgery performed by a doctor, who has less than perfect reviews.

265.   If you think, the cost of cosmetic surgery is too high in the United States, consider having the surgery done in India or Mexico. Costs are often drastically lower. You can interview doctors the same way that you would usually do, so you can expect the same level of quality work in those locations as well.

266.   Have you already checked your surgeon's school, and now you feel completely comfortable? Well, there is one more step that you should look into- malpractice. All malpractice lawsuits are available on the public record. This can help you to see if your potential surgeon, has had any past botch jobs.

267.   Make sure that the results you want to achieve from a cosmetic procedure are realistic, and not based in achieving Hollywood, red carpet perfection. There aren't always guarantees with plastic surgery. Even with the best doctor and care, you may not get the exact result you had hoped for.

268.   While it can be easy to overlook, make sure you investigate the surgery center in addition to the surgeon. The place that the procedure is going to be performed at should be licensed, or accredited. Discuss this with the doctor. If you find out that the center does not have one of these qualifications, rethink your decision to have your procedure performed there.

269.   Do some research on the location where you will be having your surgery. These places need to have a license or accreditation, and they should be inspected often. This is true when it comes to surgeon's offices as well. It is important to know that your surgery facility is up to the state's requirements and standards. If you physician is associated with a surgical center that has a questionable background, consider finding a different doctor.

270.   For any cosmetic surgery, make sure that you choose a reputable cosmetic surgeon, who has the experience to do your procedure. A great surgeon will take the time to sit down with you, and help you understand the risks involved prior to having the surgery. They will also be willing to show their credentials, and any other information that you ask for.

271.   Make sure your plastic surgeon is certified by the American Board of Plastic Surgery or the equivalent for the surgeon's home country. The websites for these agencies can quickly tell you if the surgeon in question is certified. Certification is so important because any physician can legally perform any type of medical procedure; certification ensures they've a special training in plastic surgery.

272.   Your cosmetic surgeon will make decisions that you must respect. If your doctor does not feel right doing a certain surgery on you, there is usually a good medical reason for it. If you disagree with the surgeon, get another opinion. Doing this will ensure that any surgery you have done is safer for you.

273.   It's important that you refrain from subjecting yourself to the strain of cosmetic surgery if you're in a very emotionally-fragile mental space. You need to be healthy both in body and mind to recover

from surgery. If you are not, you could be faced with complications afterwards. A slow recovery time could worsen your emotional health.

274.   Before you even have your cosmetic procedure done, it may be wise to get yourself some stool softeners. Many people experience major constipation when they have any procedure done. Plastic surgeries are no exception. Being constipated is not good for your health, a stool softener can be of great assistance.

275.   You should make yourself aware that cosmetic procedures cannot be treated as if you were shopping for a new body part. Cosmetic surgery can improve or strengthen a feature of your current physical traits, but it cannot re-do them. These procedures carry a risk with them, and you should be sure that you are 100% about the changes you are about to make to your body.

276.   Cosmetic surgery is not to be used to treat depression, or any other mental health disorders. You may get a boost of self-esteem, but if you had an underlying problem with depression, this is not going to heal that. Seek the help of a professional before, and after you have the procedure done. You'll be able to deal with the changes in a positive manner.

277.   About a month before you have your surgery, there are certain things you must take care of. Pain killers are something crucial that you need to consider. These should be stopped for at least a month before your surgery. The reason for this is that painkillers are also blood thinners. Lack of clotting will negatively affect the healing of your procedure.

278.   If you go to a second doctor for another opinion on a matter before committing to cosmetic surgery, do not tell them you have already looked into this with a prior physician. That knowledge might skew their thinking and objectivity. You want their diagnosis to be crystal clear, and to be of value to you.

279.   Make sure you understand the risks of your procedure. No medical procedure is without risks, and that includes plastic surgery. Ask your physician to explain them to you, and do your own research as well. This will help you be prepared if an unexpected negative outcome should be the result. If you are not comfortable with the level of risk you are putting yourself in, you might want to reconsider the surgery.

280.   Always do a lot of research about the cosmetic surgery clinics you are interested in. Make sure there have been no complaints against any of the surgeons who work there. If you find any complaints, you should find out exactly what happened and what the clinic did to make sure this wouldn't happen again.

281.   Do not be too embarrassed to ask your cosmetic surgeon anything you would like to know. Even if it sounds like it may be ridiculous. Having surgery is a very serious deal. You should not go through with it if, you do not understand what is involved in all aspects of the surgery.

282.   To ensure your cosmetic procedure is being being done by a trained professional, research the doctor's background. Learn where they were educated. What kinds of licenses, and certifications they have. Any extra training they may have undergone, and if there are any records of them with your local Department of Health. Also, ask the doctor how many times they've done the procedure you want.

283.   If you have heard that someone else is getting plastic surgery, don't allow that to sway your opinion of yourself. While there are many great times to use this tool, keeping up with the Jones' is

not a good enough reason. Give yourself some time to think, then reconsider the idea later on.

284.   While it can be easy to overlook, make sure you investigate the surgery center in addition to the surgeon. The place that the procedure is going to be performed at should be licensed, or accredited. Discuss this with the doctor. If you find out that the center does not have one of these qualifications, rethink your decision to have your procedure performed there.

285.   You should review the credentials of the surgeon and facility where you will be undergoing the procedure. Just as you wouldn't accept a medical practitioner without first ensuring he is capable, you shouldn't accept a clinic or hospital without knowing the details about it. This includes things such as great successes or past problems.

286.   It is very important to choose a cosmetic surgeon that has the proper certifications, to perform the procedures that you seek to get. A lot of doctors who are inexperienced in the type of service you want will offer their services to you. If you go with a doctor who has no experience, then you run the risk of the procedure not going well.

287. Remember that cosmetic surgery is indeed surgery. You are going to need recovery time when your surgery is completed. Follow your surgeon's recovery protocol exactly. This will help you feel better sooner. It will prevent infection, and further complications. Listen to your doctor's recommendations, and you will be fine.

288. If you are getting a liposuction, or a similar operation, ask your surgeon if there is anything you can do after the operation, to keep your weight down. You will probably have to get some exercise every day. Adopt a healthy diet for the effects of your surgery to last.

289. You want to do your best to find a surgeon that will be truthful and honest with you at all times. Make sure to ask about the risks involved with your procedure. If the surgeon acts like there is no possible risk and discounts your fears, you should not allow him to do your surgery.

290. Talk to your doctor about complications and risks. Make sure you understand everyone. It can be easy to be so excited that you do not consider risks or complications to your cosmetic surgery, but you have to know that they exist. Listen to your doctor and determine how you can avoid both.

291.   While you may want to enhance certain parts of your body, do not look at cosmetic surgery as a way to change the way you look in its entirety. Use it to play up your natural features, and cover up any minor flaws, that you think make you look less than beautiful.

292.   No matter what kind of plastic surgery you have had done, it is important that you protect your skin from the sun. As you may already know, UV Rays are bad for you all the time. But when you have had cosmetic surgery, it is even worse. Because your skin is already so sensitive, that the sun can quickly cause damage.

293.   Before making a decision about your plastic surgeon, ask for references. Take some time to call those references and ask them about their personal experiences. This can help you understand the quality of work that your surgeon offers, as well as the bedside manner than he or she projects to patients. Both of these things are important and should not be taken lightly.

294.   Make recovery plans at least a month in advance of your surgical procedure. Any pain medication should be considered carefully. Remember that you should abstain from painkillers during the month preceding your cosmetic procedure. This is because

pain killers can thin out your blood, resulting in worse skin repair.

295.   Prior to committing to cosmetic surgery, consider other issues that may need changing in your life. Many factors contribute to your overall appearance that will be unaffected by your surgery, so you must think about important long term lifestyle changes. Consider the possibility of changing your diet or getting help with potential depression issues.

296.   Do not be too embarrassed to ask your cosmetic surgeon anything you would like to know. Even if it sounds like it may be ridiculous. Having surgery is a very serious deal. You should not go through with it if, you do not understand what is involved in all aspects of the surgery.

297.   Compare prices among different surgeons. Don't immediately go for the cheapest price; find out what makes up the different costs. Often, the best surgeons charge the most, but assume that is always the case. You can often find a reasonably priced surgeon who does good work if you take the time to look.

298.   To ensure your cosmetic procedure is being being done by a trained professional, research the

doctor's background. Learn where they were educated. What kinds of licenses, and certifications they have. Any extra training they may have undergone, and if there are any records of them with your local Department of Health. Also, ask the doctor how many times they've done the procedure you want.

299.   Before you have a procedure done, make sure you thoroughly look into the said procedure. Many people are excited, and they rush into certain procedures. Their basic research fuels their desires. They forget to make sure that they respect the importance of such a decision, by not thoroughly research the opportunity.

300.   You should ask your surgeon what would happen if you were not satisfied with the results. If something went wrong during the procedure. Your surgeon should be honest with you. Let you know that you can file a claim for malpractice. If your surgeon is not honest on this topic, you should go to another clinic.

301.   Prevent complications from cosmetic surgery by eating a nutritious diet and using vitamin supplements when you can. Surgery is always something that takes time to get over, but you need to prepare yourself to recover by making sure your

body can do the work it needs to do. Proper nutrition will help.

302.   Check for malpractice suits before you choose a surgeon. While some malpractice suits are started frivolously, a surgeon with a history of such suits is probably a poor choice. State licensing boards, and other such local certification agencies can tell you about the malpractice history of your surgeon before you commit.

303.   Before you have surgery, validate the credentials of the surgeon. Make certain they have the education, and experience to perform the procedure. This simple step helps to ensure a positive outcome from the surgery. You should also ensure that their license, and insurance is current, and valid in your state.

304.   Before interviewing cosmetic surgeons, create a list of every question you want to ask. You need to have a good idea of a surgeon's background, and responses to critical questions. Such as questions on complications, overall risks, and post-operative care. Have the same list handy for every interview you do. You can see how each surgeon responds, and you can make an educated choice regarding the right one for you.

305.   The most important thing to consider prior to any cosmetic procedure is whether or not you actually need the surgery. Although the majority of cosmetic surgeries have positive outcomes, these procedures are not without risk. Dissatisfaction with the results, injury or even death are all possible, so it is crucial that you are certain the potential benefits outweigh the potential risks.

306.   When considering cosmetic surgery, you want to be sure that you research as much as you can about the procedure on your own. This is important, so that when you actually do talk with a professional about it the terms, and procedures that they mention are not foreign to you. That you are not hearing this information for the first time.

307.   You should make yourself aware that cosmetic procedures cannot be treated as if you were shopping for a new body part. Cosmetic surgery can improve or strengthen a feature of your current physical traits, but it cannot re-do them. These procedures carry a risk with them, and you should be sure that you are 100% about the changes you are about to make to your body.

308.   Before you go in to have cosmetic surgery, take anything you may need in your home and place it on lower shelves and out in the open. This is a good

idea because you want to stretch as little as possible after having surgery done. Straining too much can cause some damage.

309.   If you are thinking about any kind of cosmetic or plastic surgery as a smoker, you need to make an important decision. If you continue to smoke while you are in recovery, you can do real damage to your skin, resulting in ugly splotches. The choice to quit is up to you.

310.   Make sure that you do not have painted nails when you go in to have cosmetic surgery. The doctor will need to check your nails for any signs that your body is not getting enough oxygen after the anesthesia is given. Painted neails will make it nearly impossible for them to tell.

311. Be sure to consult with your primary physician first, if you are considering having cosmetic surgery done. This is usually required anyway. If you do have a condition that prevents you from safely having surgery, learn this before you spend big money consulting a plastic surgeon that you will not be able to use.